THE
BEARD BOOK
AN IDENTIFICATION AND
MAINTENANCE MANUAL OF BEARDS
AND OTHER FACE HAIR

THE
BEARD BOOK
AN IDENTIFICATION AND
MAINTENANCE MANUAL OF BEARDS
AND OTHER FACE HAIR

drawings and text
by
Ray Zimmerman

CANONGATE
Edinburgh

ISBN No. 0-914690-04-3

Library of Congress Catalog Card No. 74-81294

Published by Rampage Publishers, Danbury, Conn.

In Britain: by Canongate Publishing Ltd., 17 Jeffrey St., Edinburgh.

British ISBN No. 0-903937-09-3

Printed in the U.S.A. by The Archives Press, Danbury, Conn.

*Dedicated to Lola and others
who can't or won't.*

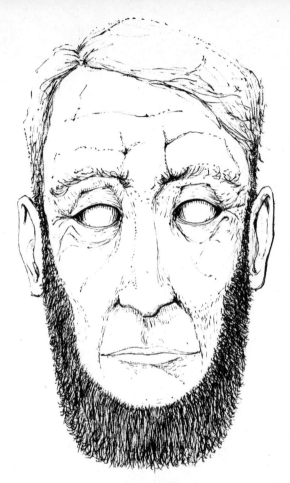

THE SWING

Conveys a depth of thought, particularly in such matters as religion and psychology. Should contrast in color with head hair. Maintenance: Constant snipping in pursuit of symmetrical curves; coloring as necessary.

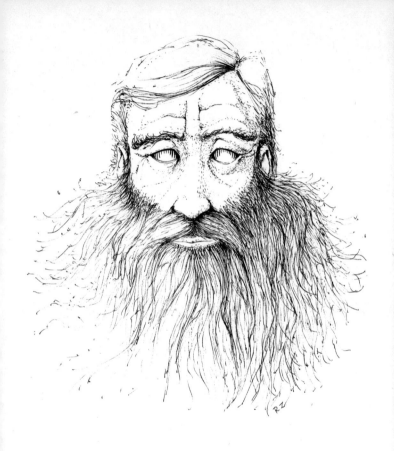

THE ROAMER

Ideal for emulating trappers. Not to be worn with zipper jacket; choice of other upper garments virtually inconsequential. Maintenance: An occasional fumigation.

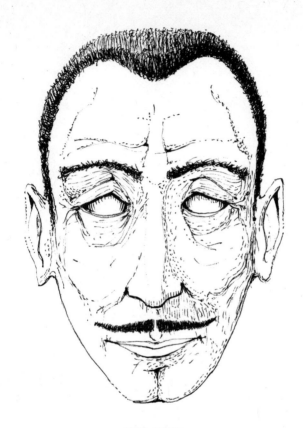

THE STRIP

Bending with slight smile, seems to work well for sales personnel in effecting closing arguments with elderly female clientele. Maintenance: Mascara and stencil, as necessary.

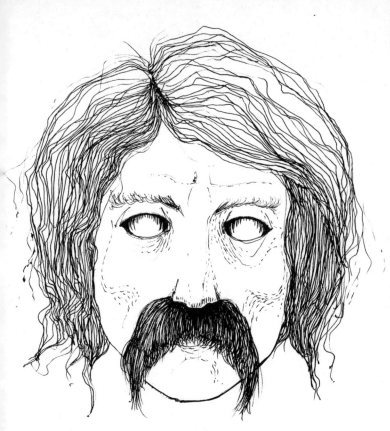

THE DROOP

Goes well with brushed denim clothing and other fake Western dress to effect a pioneer-country aspect in the midst of the modern city. Suggests a rugged, detached awareness; conceals most feelings effectively.

Maintenance: Brush, curl, snip.

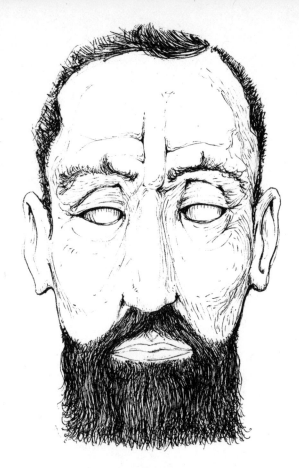

THE BLOCK

Effective with slight head hair. Presumes mysterious air, as with that of metaphysician or chess master.
Maintenance: Regular use of T square and small hedge trimmer.

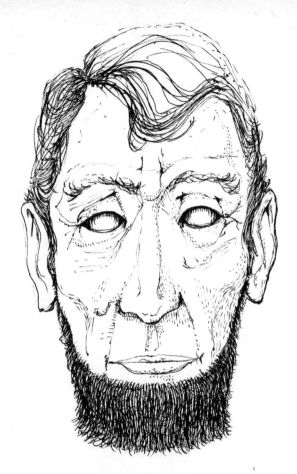

THE DEMI-BLOCK

Works best with fuller or wavier head hair. Suggests a certain historic respectability.
Maintenance: Same as for Full Block, adding slight side angles and bottom curvatures.

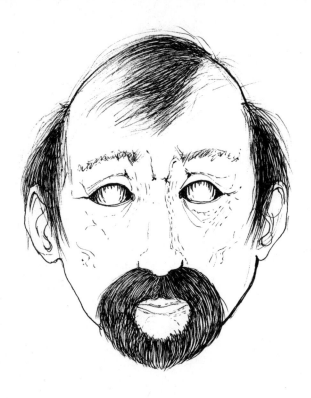

THE DOUGHNUT

Opens up the tight-lipped, thus suggesting an air of expansiveness in the ultra-inhibited. Loses effectiveness when smoking. Maintenance: Meticulous trimming, to ensure matching circumferences.

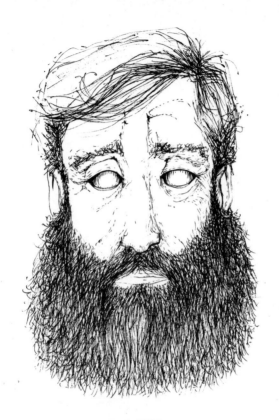

THE NEST

Recommended for middle-agers who have turned to winter sandals and summer sweaters in search of certain youth and/or intellectual disposition.
Maintenance: None.

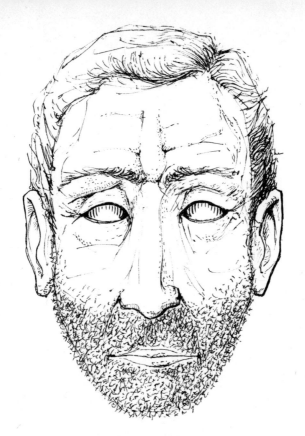

THE STARTER

Also known as The Long Weekender. Excellent for getting the general idea, when fuller growth is prohibited by job or family. Caution: Avoid loitering in public places, in consideration of local drunk tank.
Maintenance: Don't scratch.

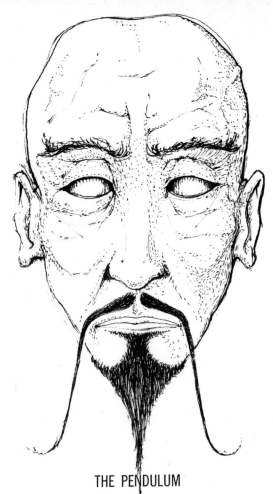

THE PENDULUM

Depends upon total baldness and ethnic particulars. Achieves a distant and mysterious appeal.

Maintenance: Thin lacquer and gentle wrist action applied daily.

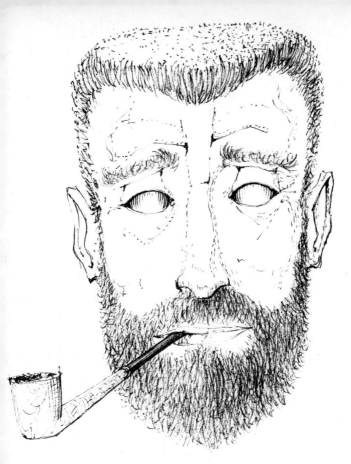

THE NOSTALGIST

Another middle-age favorite, this one conjuring notions of philoso-
phical idealism perhaps missed at an earlier age. Also popular
among advertising specialists to convey latent artistic capabilities.
Maintenance: Short, even scissors trim top and bottom. Keep an
eye on matching widow's peak and beard point.

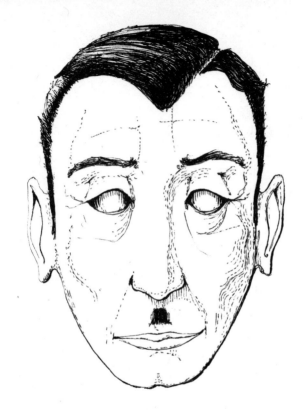

THE SPOT

Has proved most successful with those who loan money or sell antiques. Effects depend largely on delicate placement of lower facial muscles.

Maintenance: Detailed attention with tweezers and eyebrow pencil.

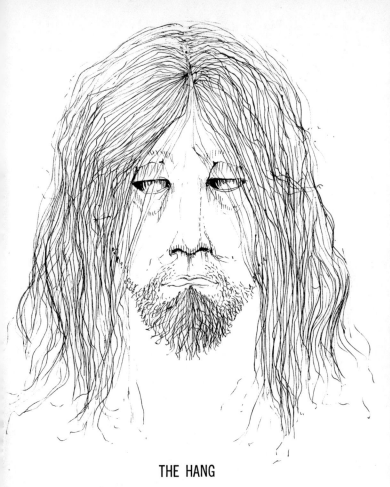

THE HANG

Depends on complete negligence of head hair. Commonly found on those in pursuit of various mystical phenomena.

Maintenance: Beard — V-trim.

Head hair — leave it alone.

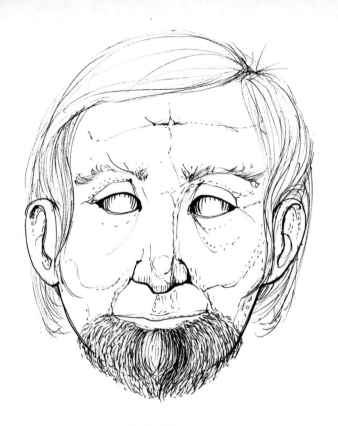

THE FEELER

For the man primarily interested in fondling himself. Requires extra-fine growth. Commonly found on elementary school teachers, marriage counselors, hotel managers and others in positions of mild authority.

Maintenance: Bathe in gentle oil, to sustain the silky touch.

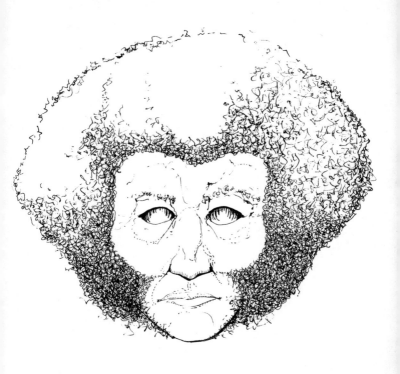

THE BAT

Has the advantage of expanding in shape, once the basic form is established. With greater volume, easily convertible to any of wide assortment of figurations, to be determined by requirements of individual wearer.

Maintenance: Shape and wait.

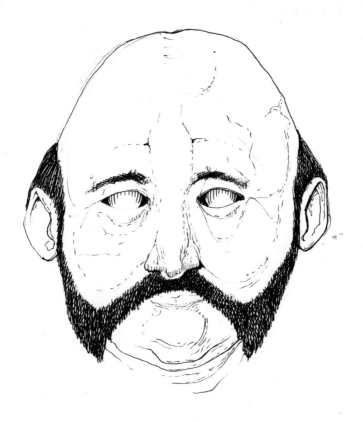

THE SNAKE

Crawls around the rear in a continuous slither. A kind of compensating ornament in which heavy stubble is kept under control and yet allowed to assert itself beyond conventional means. Maintenance: Daily and meticulous hedge work.

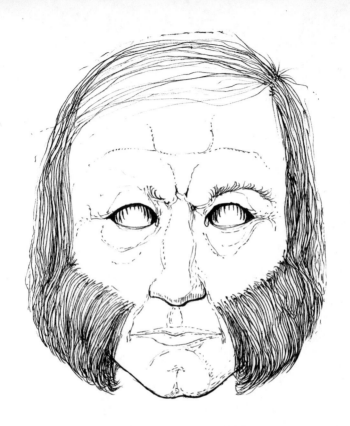

THE THREE-QUARTER CHOP

Combines the traditional with the currently fashionable. Effectively compensates for thin face or unfortunate jaw structure. Offers opportunity to display cleft.

Maintenance: Some amount of setting may be needed, depending on degree and density of growth.

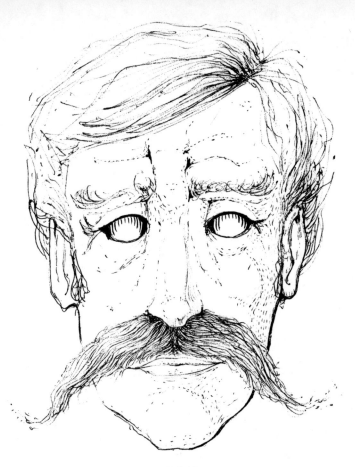

THE BAR

Suggested for those wishing to be identified with colonialism or melancholia. Accompanying waistcoat and pleated trousers, preferably in tweed, combine for best results.
Maintenance: Constant stroking, and sleeping face up.

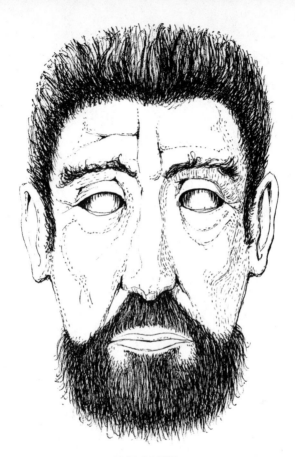

THE DRAKE

Recommended for social protestations and pursuit of abnormal pleasures. Special care urged in sustaining matching head hair texture, necessary to create overall effect.
Maintenance: Vigorous, vertical comb-pulling.

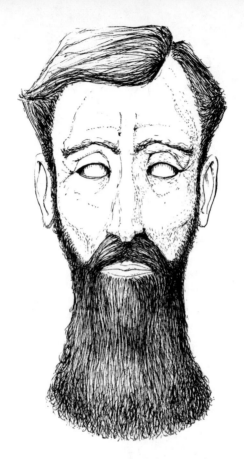

THE SMITTY

Provides certain air of iron strength. Special care must be taken to avoid slightest overlength, lest serious effect be lost completely.
Maintenance: Tie with bow at bedtime.

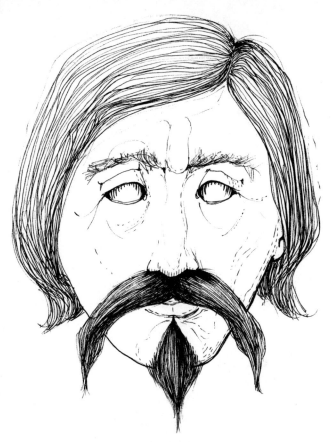

THE FORK

Recommended as a defense against ticklers and the overaffectionate. Can also be used, with practiced adroitness, as an offensive instrument.

Maintenance: Wax and stroke prongs to their sharpest.

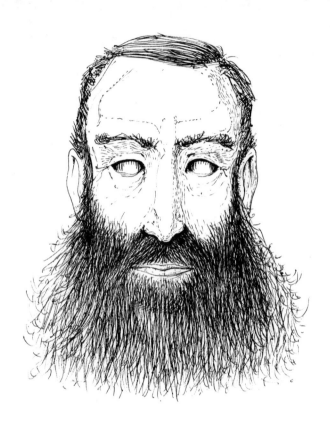

THE SAFARI

Conveys impression of perilous adventure. Most effective with military-style hat and boots. Seek widest possible extremities. Maintenance: Regular visits to vet.

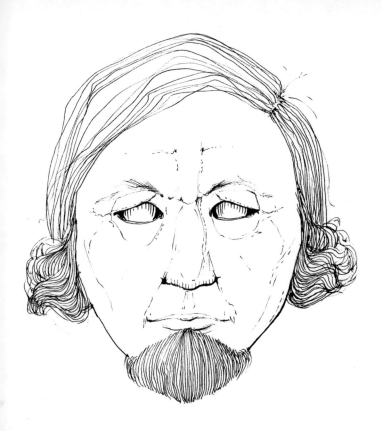

THE PATCH

Ideal for covering a weak chin or chin sore and no more. Also known as the Retarded Goatee, often seen on professors of literature who began as writers.

Maintenance: Keep curve commensurate with jaw line.

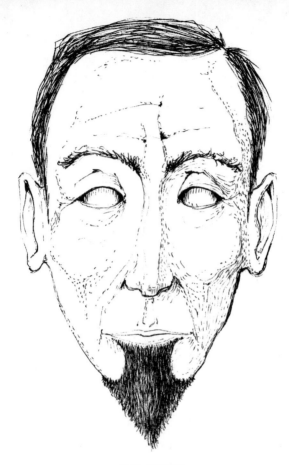

THE ARROW

Particularly recommended for dance instructors or others requiring slithery demeanor. Adapts well to ramrod physique; covers embarrassing cleft.
Maintenance: Apply ruler to sustain precise extension of jaw line.

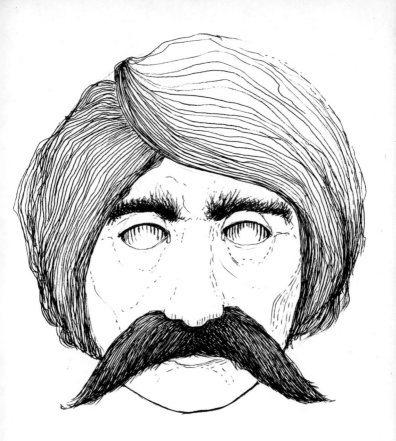

THE SUFFOCATOR

Width and style optional. The object is to inhibit breathing through the nose. For asthmatics, allergy sufferers and certain fetishists. Romantic activity may be somewhat limited.
Maintenance: Allow bush to grow well into nostrils.

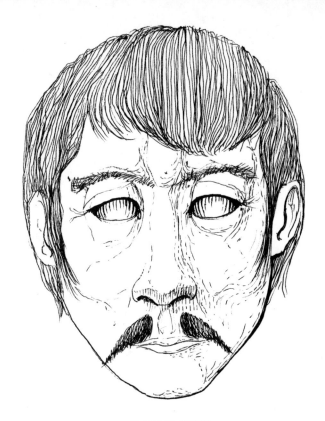

THE SPLIT SPIKE

Conveys a delicate manner. Thought to have special appeal in singles bars and at wakes. Can suggest a faint smile, so that none is actually necessary.

Maintenance: Detailed application or narrow blade razor. Angle of jut determined by direction of head hair.

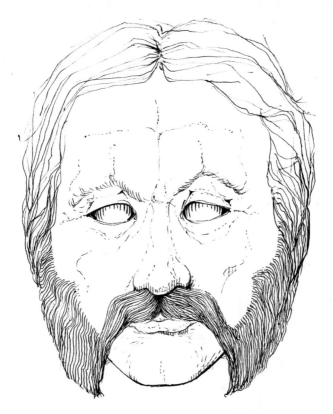

THE PRIMP

Suitable for the ultra-finicky in the art of self-adornment. Apropos for the glib and urbane, or those who need to be taken as such. Requires silky-smooth face hair.

Maintenance: Baby shampoo, gentle combing, periodic professional care.